Your Home Spa Book

How to Give Yourself an AmazingSpa
at Home

and Save Your Money

By 5K WORDS

No table of contents entries found.

Introduction

You do not need to leave your house and spend thousands of dollars at professional spa centers anymore. Now you can fully customize and create your ideal spa experience in your own home, and this book will be your step-by-step guide on how to spoil yourself with relaxing bath after a hard day's work. No longer do you need to go for the expensive chemically supplemented products in the supermarket. This book will provide you with some great skin and nails nourishing recipes that combine nature's best ingredients, most of which can be found in your kitchen.

All of this means that you no longer have to plan huge chunks of your budget for few special moments at the local spa. Now you can have an even better experience in your own bathroom, for a much smaller investment. Full body nourishing, spirit rejuvenating, completely natural spa experience in your own home on what is basically a shoestring budget? Sounds good? Let's do this!

purchaser or reader of this material. Any perceived slight, of any individual or organization is purely unintentional.

Chapter 1 - Home spa supplies

When we think of professional spa centers, the first thing that comes to our minds is cost. Most of those places are far from cheap, ironically making the whole experience somewhat stressful by itself. A stress relief place that can burn a hole in most people's budgets and leave you feeling somewhat guilty as a result? Not anymore!

Most people haven't really considered the idea of making a budget home spa, a place for relaxation and mindful, stress-free sessions for ourselves.

A shortlistcan be made, outlining the basic elements needed for a rejuvenating home spa experience.

First off, the bathtub. You need a decent size one to fill up and comfortably enjoy your precious spa moments in. Then comes a massager, which can help with blood circulation in the body and can remove built up toxins. It is an excellent addition to your home spa if your budget allows for one. An indoor water fountain can give you a more intimate experience with one of Earth's most precious elements: water. Water heals the body and the mind, and the sound effect of flowing water can be part of your home without needing to spend a fortune on building one. Pre - made, portable indoor fountains can be purchased online, and most will not a burn a whole in your budget.

For the complete home spa experience, you will want to decorate your bathroom with candles and aroma relaxing scents. You can light an aromatic candle, take a bowl of warm water and put 10 drops of your favorite essential oil inside and you have created a relaxing, natural aroma rich ambient.

Homemade or organic body lotions, shower gels, shampoos and bath salts are some of the musts - have accessories for your natural rejuvenating home spa.

Facial creams and masks containing natural foods and oils such as coconut, almond, and olive oil are very nutritious for your skin, hair and nails.

Personal nail care pedicure and manicure sets include nail files, clippers, polish, cuticle homemade cream, pedicure rasp and pumice stones for your feet.

After showering, you can wrap yourself in 100% cotton towels, warm, soft and very comfortable.

In addition, you might consider bringing plants in your bathroom as a touch of nature inside your personal space of relaxation.

Bamboo plants are very easy to find and affordable to buy, and wood relates very easily with the whole spa environment. In addition, you can buy other accessories made of wood, such as wooden hair brush, shelves and natural bamboo step mat.

Chapter 2 - Home spa bathroom decorations

The modern day model of living often brings stress, fear, anxieties, and as is the case with an increasing number of people, depression. We all need those few precious moments where all the stress and worries take a back seat and it's just us, relaxing and rejuvenating.

This makes spa & beauty centers seem like the perfect place to be for those necessary ME moments. However, the truth is, for most people these places can burn a hole in the budget, so more affordable alternatives must be considered. This is where the good news come, as with a little creativity, we can make the bathroom our magical home spa, a place where we can rejuvenate the body, the spirit and overall spoil ourselves without the luxury spa prices.

The good news is that now, with alittle effort you can transform your bathroom into your personal, soothing home spa place. When we think of such places we create a picture in our minds of soft candle light, calming scents, fluffy towels, and soothing sounds. This is something we can create for ourselves in our own homes.

It all starts with the phone, and you shut it down. In these precious moments, the last thing you need is the outside world stressing you out.

Choose your favorite ambient relaxation scents to relax your body, spirit, and mind. You can use popular scents like lavender, jasmine, peppermint or rosemary. However, you might consider choosing just one, to avoid mixing in the air. Light candles and switch off the lights for the ideal home spa ambient. Place your aromatic soaps and bath salts in a container. Feel free to place a bouquet of flowers near your tub, and if you can, consider putting up a piece of fine art on the wall. Paintings or pictures of beautiful scenery would be amazing.

Placing a bamboo plant inside your bathroom will also add a touch of exotic spa ambient for your complete relaxation and pleasure. To engage all of your sense, get a small CD player and play soothing melodies and sounds from nature. You can also play soothing spa music for the ultimate mind rejuvenation experience. A nice addition to your home spa scenery would be 100% cotton oversized fluffy towels. They will warm your body from head to toe.

Bamboo floor mats are more practical and comfortable because they allow water to vaporize faster than synthetic bath mats. Bamboo

Eco-friendly floor mats keep your bathroom cleaner and adds to the overall spa experience inside your home.

Using natural wood for your home spa adds a touch of rawness and sensation of being in direct touch with nature in your home.

Chapter 3 - Home spa tips for taking relaxing hot baths

After you have made the finishing touches on your home spa, it is time to melt away the worries and stresses by taking a long hot bath. This is the new therapeutic sanctuary you have made for yourself in your home. Pain relief, natural brain power and mood boosting, stress relief and a natural way of inducing sleep are some of the main benefits of hot, soothing baths.

First, you should take a shower, clean your body and then fill your bathtub. With a full bath tub, you can experiment with any essential oil or herb you'd like. You can also add soda or even oatmeal and some milk if you would like to go for the whole Cleopatra royal experience.

You can take care of your dry skin by adding baking soda or sea salt and 20-30 drops of jasmine or lavender essential, or any other oil of your choice.

For baby soft skin, pour 1-2 cups of full-fat milk and 1/2 cup of honey into running water, mix the ingredients and hop in. Do not forget to be fully presentin the moment. Enjoy the new home spa environment you have created for yourself. Take deep breaths and relax. Imagine the peaceful scenery and leave the world and all of your worries behind.

Honey contains high levels of antioxidants, is moisturizing, softening and detoxing 100% natural product. Full-fat milk is very exfoliating and gives the skin a calming effect. When you finish with this relaxation technique, take a warm shower to rinse the honey and milk from your skin.

Consider soaking your body in a mixture of water and salt, especially Epsonsalt, which is great after a workout or a stressful busy day. Salt is an excellent ingredient to mix with water as it contains lots of magnesium, which the body needs and absorbs. It can also be used for curing different types of, skin conditions, as well for detoxing and relaxation purposes.

While the water is filling the tub, put 20-30 drops of your favorite essential oil and your shower gel. Eucalyptus helps with sinus problems, Rosemary essential oil is great for relaxation and clarity. The use of aromatic essential oils gave rise to aromatherapy, a therapeutic process based on the medicinal properties of oils that can soothe and cure certain health conditions.

Taking herbal baths for healing and relaxation.

To treat yourself with an herbal bath, you probably don't even have to visit the local store for dried herbs. Most of the materials you need can be found in your kitchen.

Brew 1 liter of tea and add 10-15 drops of essential oil of your choice. You should use stronger tea, such as green tea for energizing or chamomile and peppermint tea for relaxation and calming sensation. You are good to go. Enjoy yourself.

Natural bath salts

2 cups of Epsom salt

2 teaspoons of fruit oil of your choice

5-10 drops of your favorite essential oil

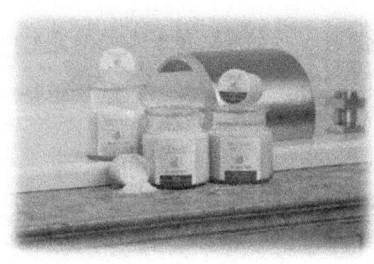Optional: a drop of two of liquid food coloring

1/4 cup sea salt

1 tablespoon of baking soda

Mix the ingredients well with a spoon and leave it in a jar. Use it when you are having a hot bath to fully enjoy your intimate relaxation moments.

Chapter 4 - Home spa natural products for healthy and younger-looking skin

You don't need to pay a fortune to have your skin naturally healthy glowing and nourished. Nature provides us with ingredients that are very effective and affordable. The following recipes will nourish, heal and protect your body.

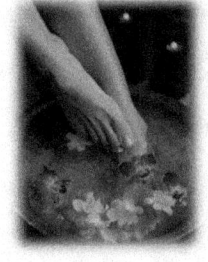 Make a body butter recipe:

Coconut oil (1/2 cup)

Olive or castor oil (1 tsp)

AloeVera gel (2 tsp)

And you can use lime or lavender oil.

Mix the ingredients together with an electric mixer for 5 minutes and spoon the butter into a glass jar. This can be stored in a refrigerator or kept at a room temperature.

Egg - face mask

The egg is one of the healthiest and nutritional foods we have.

Mix 1 raw egg with 1 tps of honey together and apply on your face and neck.Keep it there for 15 minutes and then rinse with warm water.

For rough hand skin, you only need 2-3 cups of warm milk. The fat from the milk will hydrate your hands and vitamin E will nourish your dry skin.

Baking soda or sea salt for tired feet.

Add 1/2 cup of baking soda and pure vanilla or lavender essential oil in a tub with warm water. Lay back and enjoy the beautiful sensation, feeling the relaxation coming up your feet.

You can also do this with 1/4 cup of sea water and 15-20 drops of your favorite essential oils.

There is a natural remedy for eye wrinkles and all you need is 3 tablespoons of raw milk and the same quantity of honey. Mix the two ingredients over a gentle fire and apply the warm mixture around the eyes. After 30 minutes, you can rinse it off with warm water.

For the ideal natural solution for acne, mix together 2 tbsp of baking soda, 1/2 cup of lemon juice, 5 tbsp honey and 1tbps cinnamon powder. Apply the mixture on your face, and after 5 minutes you can wash it off with warm water.

Natural homemade hair removal wax

All the ingredients you need for this recipe can be found in your kitchen. No need to spend that extra money on a visit to a local saloon or on an expensive hair removal wax from the cosmetics store. All you need is some sugar, lemon, and water.

2 cups of white sugar

3/4 cups water

2 tsp lemon juice

Combine the ingredients in a saucepan and heat it on a low temperature. The mixture will thicken and turn golden brown.

Stir the mixture to make sure that all the sugar is dissolved. When it becomes golden, pour it into a stainless steel bowl.

While the wax is cooling, you can exfoliate your body and have the satisfaction of knowing that you are using a recipe containing all natural ingredients that are easy on the budget.

Once the natural wax cools down enough, take part of it with a spoon, roll it into a ball and knead the mixture until it becomes smooth. Then you can apply it on your skin in the direction your hair grows, not against it.

You can use this wax for facial hair, arm and leg hair. What is left of the mixture can be reused later. All you need to do is put it in a microwave for a couple of minutes and you are good to go.

Natural, fast and simple.

Coffee, sugar and olive oil for perfect smooth skin.

Coffee is rich in antioxidants and contains vitamin E. It also helps you get rid of cellulite. Mixed with sugar and olive oil, it can be used for thorough deep skin baths for removing dead skin.

For best results, you can repeat this process after every shower you take.

Cooling peppermint foot cream

14 cups Shea Butter

1/4 cup Coconut Oil

2 Tablespoons Olive Oil

15 drops Peppermint essential oil

Combine Shea butter and coconut oil on a gentle fire and stir the ingredients for about a minute. Once the ingredients melt and combine nicely, leave the mixture to cool down for 5 minutes and then add olive and peppermint essential oil.

For best application, consider using socks before going to bed.

Chapter 5- Homespa treatments for healthy and strong nails

While you're giving yourself home spa treatments and reading hope spa tips, you can also give your nails professional salon quality manicure and pedicure. The first step towards getting your perfect nails is removing the old nail polish. After that, gently file them into shape before soaking your hands and feet in warm water. Filing should be done in one direction only, as to avoid damaging your nails. Soak your hands and feet in a tub filled with warm water. You can add shower gel, baking soda, and essential oils of your choice. Jasmine essential oil is great for relaxation and peppermint oil is excellent for acooling sensation. These ingredients will soften your nails, remove the dead skin cells and the essential oils will moisturize your skin.

Make a homemade scrub to soften your feet, remove dead cells and rejuvenate the skin.

Mix 2 tablespoons of sugar, 1 tsp lemon juice and 1 tablespoon of honey. In addition, you can consider including 1 tablespoon of coconut or almond essential oil and a bowl filled with warm water. The ingredients should be well mixed and then you can scrub your feet using acircular motion. After this, you can wash your hands and feet with cold water.

You can use coconut/olive/almond/Argan oil to apply to your nails and cuticles and leave it for 5-10 minutes. After that, you can wipe off the oils and gently push back the cuticles. Apply a base coat and then paint on two thin layers of your favorite nail color.

Use vitamin E to moisturize and hydrate your brittle nails. Apply it before going to sleep and massage gently, as this helps with circulation. Do this on a daily basis. Sea salt can also help with damaged nails and provide a touch of aesthetics with a fresher, shinier look.

Mix 1tablespoons of sea water and oils of your choice and soak your nails in the mixture for 15 minutes. Do this 3 -4 times per week for ideal results.

Nail growth

Horsetail tea for strong nail growth

The horsetail herb is full of minerals, calcium, and silica. You can use this herb to encourage better nail growth.

After you have prepared horsetail tea for yourself, wait for it, cool down and then soak your nails in it for 20 minutes. Do this several times a week for best results.

Almond hand nail cream recipe

Homemade hand cream can save you money and will help you avoid applying factory produced cosmetics on your skin. This cream will protect your nails and the skin on your hands. To make this great recipe at home prepare the following ingredients:

1/4 cup of beeswax

1/2 cup of almond oil

1/2 cup of coconut oil

1/4 cup of rosewater

Melt beeswax and add the almond and coconut oil including rosewater and stir until your homogeneous mixture. Pour it into a container and leave it to cool naturally. Use this cream applying it to your fingernails with a gentle massage.

Egg soaks recipe for strong and healthy nails

For this awesome recipe, you will need to prepare

2egg yolks

1/4 cup of milk

1tbs honey

Mix the ingredients well and soak your nails for 15 minutes and rinse well.

Another healthy nutritional recipe consisting of natural ingredients is the mixture of lemon juice and Argan oil. Ideally you should soak your nails in the mixture for 20 minutes, or you can even apply the mixture to your nails using cotton and leave it overnight.

Chapter 6 - Home-spa recipe treatments for a marvelous healthy hair

Hair care starts with the scalp skin, so in order to improve the health of our hair, we must not neglect the health of our scalp. Nutritious, healthy ingredients that will make your hair strong, beautiful and silky smooth can be found in your kitchen. A very simple, yet effective ingredient for natural, shiny hair is tea. Warm, unsweetened, and ideally, about one litter of it should be applied to your hair after showering. As tea can have hair coloring properties, we must be careful which tea we use. Black tea is generally recommended for brunettes while chamomile tea is ideal for blondes. You can apply this every time after washing your hair, as a final touch without fear of side effects.

A highly effective recipe for damaged hair is the apple cider vinegar mask. You should mix 1 tsp apple cider vinegar, 2 tsp olive oil, and 3 egg whites. Rub this mix into your hair for about 30 min, and then shampoo and rinse. Make your hair grow faster naturally by applying to it a litter of warm nettle leaves tea. Again, you can do this after every hair wash.

Home remedies for hair loss.

There are many people suffering from hair loss nowadays, and age, stress, medical conditions, genes and chemically enriched hair products are just some of the factors behind it. There are oils which you can use by applying them to your hair, that will slow down the unpleasant process of hair loss. The list includes argan oil, coconut or almond oil, castor oil and wheat germ oil. For added effect include 5-10 drops of rosemary essential oil, and again, the correct application technique is a gentle massage from the root to the tip of your hair. You should do this at least once a week.

Make your own anti-dandruff shampoo using nothing but natural ingredients

3 tsp Aloe Vera gel

1 tsp baking soda

1 tsp lemon juice

Mix the ingredients well and pour into a clean bottle. You now have your own anti-dandruff homemade shampoo that can also make your hair soft and silky.

Coconut lavender hair conditioner

1 cup coconut oil

1 teaspoon vitamin E oil

1 teaspoon jojoba oil

5 drops lavender essential oil

Pour all the ingredients in a bowl and mix using an electric mixer for about a minute. Then you can pour it into a container. After washing your hair take some of the mixture and gently apply it on your hair. Leave it there for 20 minutes and then rinse it off with warm water.

The conditioner will help you with split ends and leave your hair strong, healthy and silky smooth.

One of the best natural hair tools is simply a wooden hairbrush. These brushes naturally condition your hair without producing static electricity, massage the scalp and improve the blood circulation. Also, wooden brushes deal with hair tangles easily when the hair is wet. Nature can be truly amazing.

Chapter 7 - Gifts from sea for health and beauty of your body

Recipe #1.

This recipe will perfectly solve problems of rough or chapped skin.

Sea salt has a strongly marked crystal structure. Therefore, instead of applying a scrub, salt will serve your skin get rid of dead skin flakes and make it easy and placid. Just rub a fine sea salt with light circular movements, at the same time, try to avoid skin face or damaged skin. Salt perfectly heals old wounds, but eat away fresh one. In addition, you should be more conscious about using salt if you have sensitive skin.

If you want to use sea salt instead of the scrub for the face, mix a small pinch of salt with a small amount of neutral soap to the consistency of paste. Then apply it on the face and with smooth and soft massaging movements rub into the skin, avoiding the areas around the eyes. This scrub cleans the pores from dust and dirt and allows skin to breath better. Since salt is in crystal form do scrub

Gently to avoid scratching the skin. Do purification process for a few minutes, then rinse with cool water or an infusion of chamomile, sage, mint. Be sure to put on a face moisturizer or nourishing cream. For deep cleansing I recommend pre-steam the face, holding it over the steam. You can use all the same aforementioned infusions of herbs.

Lighter scrubs and Exfoliants, where the salt is the primary, but not the main ingredient. For example, salt scrubs from Ahava, and Guam. Any products can supplement such care, which includes a moisturizing oil. You can use baby oil from Johnson & Johnson. This purification process, beauticians recommend to carry out 1-2 times a week for oily and combination skin; 1-2 times a month for normal, dry and sensitive skin.

Recipe #2.

The following recipe can get rid of pimples and blackheads.

The reason for their appearance is clogging the pores. Use toners and cleansers, containing marine ingredients. You can make a mask of mud or clay that perfectly cleanses, opens the pores and improves blood circulation. In addition, sea mud and algae facilitate to the elimination of toxins and impurities, thereby improving skin condition and complexion color. You can use the seaweed - kelp, which are sold in dry form in a pharmacy or specialized funds. For these dilute algae with water heated to fifty degrees. Let stand for an hour, and then put it on the face as a mask. The procedure lasts 20-30 minutes. The recipe is also suitable for the entire body. You only need to increase the amount of algae: a bucket of water, add four packs of algae, let it stand for long, strain and apply the mask on the body. Then it is best to wrap yourself up in a sheet and lay down for an hour or more. If you suffer from allergies, it is better to check first reaction of the skin to such compress.

To energize or cleanse the skin of the body you can use seaweed baths. To do this, put the algae in fabric bag (well transmitting water) and place it in a bath during a set of water. Such bath will not only effectively affect the condition of your skin, but also will bring relief to tired muscles and will relax. To avoid allergies when buying cosmetics, try a small amount at first to try to find out whether your body negative reactions.

Recipe #3.

This advice is suitable for "tired" skin, which lost glow, for withering and aging skin.

Arouse internal resources to return the skin to life and enhance the metabolism are quite capable for the treasures of the seas and oceans. The composition of many cosmetic series include seaweed (brown, blue, green, red), extracts from the skin and fins of fish, plankton, coral, shells, concentrated sea water and some minerals. Creams, which include these resources, are suitable for all skin types and for all ages. The company Thalgo - one of the most interesting companies in our country is actively working with the gifts of the sea.

Recipe #4.

If you are unhappy with the appearance of your legs the hated cellulite, swelling, excessive wrinkles, use the accompanying formula. Above all, it is worth mentioning that doctors not without reason called legs the "second heart". From a good blood, circulation in the veins of the legs depends blood circulation in the whole body. Of course, marine cosmetics will help to reach a stable, positive effect, simply without a balanced diet and exercise; still the problem cannot be resolved. Cosmetics are a good helper in the fight against cellulite.

Beach Resort - a great tool in the fight against the problems, many beauty salons, experts recommend arranging it at home 1-2 times a week. Dissolve in a water bath (38 ° C) 40 grams of powdered algae or 100 g of sea salt with algae. These products you can find in stores that sell cosmetics and health products or in pharmacies. Soak in such bath for 20 minutes. Throw with a bathrobe, but do not rinse or return to Terry sheets and relax for 20 minutes (at the same time you can energize the face with a mask from algae). Just after that takes a cool shower and rub anti-cellulite cream.

One of the cheapest and, most important, effective methods of prevention of cellulite - baths with essential oil of lemon. Under the shower, thoroughly rub the problem areas with a massage glove or rough washcloth to light redness. Dissolve in the bath one-kilogram sea salt and add 4-5 drops of lemon essential oil - sold in pharmacies, cosmetic stores. Enjoy 20 minutes. Then rub anti-cellulite cream or gel.

Microelements, which are part of sea salt, can normalize metabolic process in cells. Under their effect will accumulate less fluid, fats will start to actively break down, that will eventually lead to a visible improvement in the figure.

In addition to the baths, use anti-cellulite creams, gels and lotions from the Clarins Company and, of course, products for Nivea.

If, because you have a lot of walking, standing or sitting at work, you have tired legs or you are worried about dry skin, with the help hasten the gifts from the depths of the sea. Try products of seaweed, which exfoliate dead skin cells, nourish and hydrate it. These products will help to make your skin smooth, soft and silky. The same applies to the sea salt with micronized algae.

Try milk oil for the bath, toning shower gel with sea minerals from Nivea, oil from the Matis or products of known companies Thalgo and Biotherm.

Contrast baths - hot with sea salt or algae, or cool with chamomile essential oils - the ideal way not only to relieve fatigue and swelling of the legs, but also to improve blood circulation.

It is useful once to pamper your legs with following procedures once a week.

Baths:

- Contrasting (possible with common salt or sea salt)
- improves blood circulation 5 minutes in hot 1

minute in cold water. Increase the process up to 2 times

- Chamomile, mint - reduce sweating and fatigue 6 tablespoons. l. Chamomile (mint), stand for 1 hour in 2 liters of boiling water, drain, heat, keep your feet until the water will cool;

- With ice cubes and menthol - relieves swelling

- Calendula - for cracked skin prevention fungal diseases: pour 1 tbsp. OfCalendula with 1 liter of boiling water.

You can try a procedure, which is widely used in the spa: lower leg in a warm marine mud, then put on socks (not wool). Keep mud mask for legs for 1 hour.

Recipe #5.

If you do not like dull hair with split ends, use this recipe.

Hair suffer mostly in summer, especially if you spend a vacation on the beach. Sea salt - is a direct threat to the hair. However, oddly enough, to this issue, you can apply the expression "fight fire with fire." All the same, marine product – algae will come to help your hair. Many hairdresser experts affirm that to moisturize and strengthen the hair, as well as to make them shine; the most suited are products containing extracts of kelp.

It is more convenient to use ready-made shampoos, but you can rinse hair in infusion of the dried seaweed soaked in water. Pay attention to the cosmetic series "Spa at home" - the company Ahava.

The Dead Sea – is a unique and natural source of beauty and health. Salts and Dead Sea mudused for long for medicinal purposes. Magical cosmetic properties of minerals of the Dead Sea have been well-known since the days of the Egyptian Queen Cleopatra.

Natural minerals in its unique combination, which is doing magic with the skin: cleanse, nourish, tone and maintain the required level of moisture. Ahava - the only in the world cosmetic, which is produced from beginning to end on the shores of the Dead Sea. The result of applying this cosmetic is noticeable within a few days: the skin is firmer, smoother and younger looking, as after a holiday in the resort.

How to use algae at home

When you sweat in the bath or sauna, many different toxins that have collected in your subcutaneous fat and blood, are allocated through the pores. Detoxifying bath with baking soda, English or sea salt can also help remove toxins from your body. Sit in the bath up to 20 minutes, and then gently rub the skin with a soapy brush made of natural fibers, such as pig bristle, dry brush or mitten of loofah. Try to rub the dry skin with a brush - is an ancient healing method that was used in ancient centuries to enhance blood circulation and lymph circulation. Massage your body once a day with a brush made of natural bristles, which you can buy in health stores. Massage with short, jerky movements for better effect, toward the heart. Seaweed body wrap - a revitalizing, toning and activating cell procedure that will revitalize and improve the tone of your skin. Use wakame seaweed (or any, which you will find).

Fresh seaweed should be briefly immersed in warm water, then rinse to remove salt. The dried wakame should be immersed in water for 20 minutes to get soften. After you have thoroughly cleaned the skin, put strips of seaweed all over the body. Then lie down for 30 minutes. Remove algae, rinse with cold water.

Cleansing the face and body before wrapping algae:

Gather hair into a bun, so face and neck will be visible. Apply on your hand more cleansing lotion. Lightly pound and put it on the neckline, neck and face.

Carefully wipe the skin with soft circular moves to remove cosmetics and dust (you can use a cotton swab).

For compress, pour hot water in medium capacity. Moisten in it a small towel, wring and put it on your face. Lightly press it and keep breathing evenly and deeply. Remove compress and repeat the procedure.

Spray the face with thermal water to neutralize the effect of limewater to the skin. With wet fingertips, apply creamy scrub with algae to the skin and massage. Constantly moisten your fingers. Remove the scrub using a compress.

For body scrub, take a handful of sea salt mixed with oil. You can use this mixture putting it a fabric bag. Apply the mixture on the body and rinse off in the shower with massaging moves. Sea salt revitalizes your skin and prepares it to absorb nutrients from the algae. It is important - as the scrub contains oil, to put on the floor in the bathroom rubber mat, so you would not slip.

Algae wraps:

Take a bag of algae and add a little water to make a paste. Spread one of the pieces of aluminum foil in the bath, the second put ready nearby. In addition, put the garbage bag next to the bath.

• Wear disposable gloves and apply a paste of seaweed on the entire body: first shoulders and back – as far as you can reach, then on the legs, abdomen, and finally on arms. All this, of course, is quite tiring process, but the result is worth the trouble.

• Carefully sit in the bath on the foil and cover with the second piece. You will be warm enough so you get into some kind of pressure chamber. The body temperature will rise, the skin pores will open and algae start to have an effect.

• Lay like that about half an hour.

• Fold the foil and immediately put it in a garbage bag. Thoroughly rinse the algae with water in the shower. It will be the best if you will use bath mitt. In addition, cold shower, in the conclusion, will strengthen the body.

• Algae great rids the body of toxins and return skin elasticity. If you will massage problematic areas with a special cream, the effect of algae will be even stronger.

Conclusion

Putting in the time and effort to create a special home spa experience for yourself in your own home will prove to be a worthy investment in the long run. Having your own escape from the world, the stress relief day is simply priceless.

Putting together something like this says that you appreciate and respect yourself first. We all deserve some quality me - time, alone with our thoughts at the end of the day, in the perfect rejuvenating environment of our own creation. A place that will heal your mind, body and spirit, and prepare you for new challenges ahead.

With such thorough and deep therapeutic treatments provided using nature's best resources, your happiness will skyrocket. You will be more relaxed and positive and full of energy

You will also feel younger and stronger in spirit, no matter how old you are. Reconnect with Nature, for it is the best way to rejuvenate and reclaim your inner strengths and balance in life.